I0486712

Metabolic Syndrome

The Ultimate Cure Guide for How to Fix Your Metabolic Syndrome Once and for All

presentation of the information is without contract or any type of guarantee assurance.

The trademarks that are used are without any consent, and the publication of the trademark is without permission or backing by the trademark owner. All trademarks and brands within this book are for clarifying purposes only and are owned by the owners themselves, not affiliated with this document.

Table Of Contents

Introduction

You've probably heard about "Metabolic Syndrome" at some point. Maybe you've heard about how it has affected millions of people around the globe or maybe you've heard that it has been growing at a rapid pace. So, what exactly is metabolic syndrome and what can we do about it?

This short and concise book will focus on the history of metabolic syndrome, the science behind it, the symptoms, and how it can affect one's body. Most practically, we will look at the ways to diagnose metabolic syndrome, along with the major prevention and treatment options.

In this book we are aiming to educate you on this topic in an unbiased light. If you feel like you may have metabolic syndrome after reading this, make sure to see your doctor right away.

We hope that you are able to learn a thing or two from reading this!

Chapter 1:

What is Metabolic Syndrome?

Metabolic syndrome refers to any disorder affecting the metabolic functions. This is mainly reflected as a defect of energy utilization and storage, leading to unwanted effects and a higher propensity for specific diseases. Considered a "disease of affluence," incidences of this condition are significantly higher in developed countries. For instance, it is estimated that 34% of the United States population has metabolic syndrome.

At the same time, people become more prone to this disease as they advance in age. This is partly due to the natural decline in digestive/metabolic function as a person advances in age. Metabolic syndrome is also known as Syndrome X, cardio-metabolic syndrome, insulin resistance syndrome, and Reaven's syndrome.

There are five medical conditions that medical professionals look at when trying to diagnose and characterize metabolic syndrome. As a rule of thumb, having three or more of these signs will yield a positive diagnosis. These are:

Abdominal Obesity

This is the main indicator of metabolic syndrome. This is primarily characterized as being overweight and having excessive fat accumulation around the waist and trunk. This fat, instead of accumulating beneath the skin or interspersed with muscles, deposit at the peritoneal cavity, leading to the buildup of so-called "visceral fat." At the time of this publication, standards regarding abdominal obesity tend to differ from one authority to another.

However, it is mostly agreed upon that having a waist circumference above 40 inches for men and 35 inches for women is an affirmative sign of abdominal obesity. Body mass index (BMI) is also useful in evaluating if a person has abdominal obesity.

High Blood Pressure

Termed as hypertension, this medical condition is characterized by an elevated arterial blood pressure. High blood pressure usually refers to chronic hypertension, as even healthy individuals can experience acute hypertension during moments of physical activity or stress.

A person is diagnosed with hypertension when their blood pressure is persistently at or above 140/90. When left unchecked, this can increase the risk of developing cardiovascular diseases such as myocardial infarction, coronary heart disease, strokes, aneurysms, and kidney failure.

High Fasting Plasma Glucose

This is a condition where there is an excessive amount of glucose present in blood plasma. A person's fasting glucose level serves as a more accurate diagnostic modality for hyperglycemia, as being in a fed state significantly alters serum glucose levels. People with fasting blood glucose levels between 100 and 125 mg/dl are hyperglycemic, while those who have readings that go beyond 125 mg/dl are positive for diabetes mellitus. A chronic increase in plasma glucose can cause significant damage in multiple organs.

High Serum Triglycerides

This is a condition characterized by elevated levels of triglyceride in the blood. Triglycerides are the most common forms of fat molecules found in the human body, but an excess of these in the bloodstream can lead to health problems such as atherosclerosis. Usually asymptomatic, such a condition is often diagnosed only after blood tests or when a complication that has already surfaced. Having triglyceride levels over 200 mg/dl is a positive indicator of high triglyceride levels. Those with triglyceride levels between 150-200 mg/dl would be considered "under observation."

Low High-Density Lipoprotein

The level of high-density lipoprotein, also termed as HDL, is generally considered to be one of the best ways to evaluate cardiovascular health. This is because an increased level of HDL in blood serum lowers the odds of lipids depositing in the arterial walls, which leads to atherosclerosis. Essentially, this is because HDL functions as a means for transporting lipids away from tissues and into the liver for processing. A person has low high-density lipoprotein if their HDL levels go below 40 mg/dl for men and 50 mg/dl for women.

There are other ways to evaluate a patient for metabolic syndrome (will be discussed at a later part of this book), but these five parameters are the primary determining factors for diagnosis. This means that you may have one of these and not be considered for metabolic syndrome. However, having all (or most) of these conditions means that you have this condition. At the same time, you will become more prone to all the complications associated with it, such as cardiovascular disease and diabetes.

Chapter 2:

History of Metabolic Syndrome

The history of metabolic syndrome and diabetes mellitus are fundamentally intertwined with each other. The idea that a pathologic condition (or more like a set of pathologic conditions) that increases one's propensity for having diabetes already existed as early as the 1920's. While the term "metabolic syndrome" came much later, the fact that physicians and scientists were already doing their investigations for this condition means that there was clearly something lying underneath the surface.

The French doctor, Jean Vague, made a groundbreaking finding that led to the eventual "discovery" of the metabolic syndrome in 1947. Observing both his patients and available clinical data, Vague deduced that upper body obesity predisposes patients to a variety of diseases, including diabetes, atherosclerosis, kidney stones and gout. Around the same time, a research team led by

Avogadro and Crepaldi observed that a hypocaloric, low-carbohydrate diet, helped moderately obese patients recover from diabetes and lower their serum cholesterol and triglyceride levels.

It was in 1977 when the term "metabolic syndrome" was first publicly used. Herman Haller coined the term while studying risk factors associated with diabetes. This mainly served as a reference to the complex associations between obesity, diabetes, hyperlipidemia, increased uric acid levels and fatty liver disease. He also studied the potential contributing effects of the aforementioned conditions to the development of atherosclerosis.

People such as Gerald B. Phillips, by combining other health issues such as hyperlipoprotenemia and myocardial infarction, further expanded such associations. Phillips, in particular, proposed the possibility that the identification of a linking factor between these different health conditions could provide the key to preventing cardiovascular disease.

In 1988, Gerald M. Reaven, using his Banting lecture as a jumping point, made the hypothesis that insulin resistance is the central linking factor that connected the signs and effects of metabolic syndrome together. He termed the combination of all these abnormalities "Syndrome X," with each increasing a person's propensity to develop type 2 diabetes and cardiovascular ailments linked to atherosclerosis.

Since then, numerous research projects have been conducted in order to try and uncover potential answers to counter the spread of metabolic syndrome. Meanwhile, the frequency of occurrence of this condition is still rising steadily. If there is a positive from that disturbing news, then an increased awareness caused a conscious effort from both the general public and local governing bodies to make preventive efforts to stop the further progression of this disease.

At the same time, "cures" were created to keep metabolic syndrome and its end effects in check. The fight of the medical community to reduce cases of metabolic syndrome, obesity, diabetes, and cardiovascular disease is still ongoing and far from over.

Chapter 3:

The Science Behind Metabolic Syndrome

To better understand how metabolic syndrome affects the body, it is important to take a closer look at the science regarding how the disease develops. To better answer this, it is important to take a look at the pathophysiology behind the development and progression of this disease. With a better understanding on how the disease works, one can better understand how to prevent and potentially resolve this syndrome.

The best way to begin here is to review the five main risk factors associated with metabolic syndrome: abdominal obesity, high blood pressure, high fasting glucose levels, high serum triglycerides, and low HDL levels. As mentioned earlier, when at least three out of these five conditions are present, it means that the patient is positive for metabolic syndrome and is at a higher risk of developing type 2 diabetes and cardiovascular disease, almost by default.

Arguably, the biggest risk factor associated with the development of metabolic syndrome is the accumulation of visceral fat. In many ways, health experts believe that fat accumulated in the abdomen is significantly more harmful than fat deposited underneath the skin (called subcutaneous fat). This is mainly because visceral fat poses a lot of negative threats to the human body.

For example, visceral fat can trigger increased levels of plasma TNFA, a chemical compound linked to both the formation of inflammatory cytokines and the development of insulin resistance. Also, increased visceral fat leads to an increase in immune cells, which leads to increased inflammation. Chronic inflammation is linked to hypertension, atherosclerosis, and diabetes.

An increased consumption of excess sugar and fat, especially if such chronic overconsumption is done simultaneously, is directly linked to the development of metabolic syndrome. This has been shown in a number of animal research studies. The excess fat ingested in the diet, combined with the excess carbohydrates converted into fat, leads to the marked increase in triglyceride levels in the blood. Increased levels of triglycerides means a significant increase in one's risk factors for developing atherosclerosis.

This risk is further increased if the patient has low HDL and high LDL, as more of these fats end up getting deposited in large blood vessels, such as the coronary arteries. Aside from this, excess fat is converted into arachidonic acid. As the precursor of prostaglandins and leukotrienes, this acid triggers the formation of inflammatory factors.

A chronic increase in blood glucose levels is one of the pinpointed causes of type 2 diabetes. This is something that is routinely observed in causes of metabolic syndrome. The mechanism behind this slow yet constant process of blood sugar elevation is pretty straightforward. Consuming excessive amounts of carbohydrates over long periods of time will cause the eventual elevation of blood glucose levels.

Aside from that, some of this excess would be transformed into fat, with some or even most of that fat ending up stored at the viscera. Once developed, it then triggers the cascade of effects that lead to diabetes, insulin resistance, and cardiovascular damage.

As you can tell by now, a complex list of predisposing factors causes the development of metabolic syndrome. This is because the alteration of multiple biological processes triggers the syndrome. Sure, correlating one or even two of the main symptoms involved in this syndrome is relatively easy, but condensing all these elaborate pathways within a singular structure does not suffice.

Here are some causes and risk factors associated with metabolic syndrome. Having any of these makes you more prone to the disease. Just like the five fundamental signs, having more of these potential causes makes you more prone to developing metabolic syndrome.

Age

A person will become more prone to developing metabolic syndrome as he/she advances in age. This trend is observed regardless of race, gender, or social level. In fact, metabolic syndrome is reportedly observed in around 40% of all individuals above the age of 60. This is because aging naturally affects multiple aspects of human metabolism, making aged people more prone to the type of health decline associated with metabolic syndrome.

Stress

Chronic exposure to stress is one of the leading causes of disease development. The same holds true with metabolic syndrome. This is mainly because stress has the ability to disrupt the function of the hypothalamus-pituitary-adrenal axis. With this critical endocrine pathway compromised, cortisol production is increased, leading to an increase in glucose and insulin levels. This promotes the accumulation of visceral fat, insulin resistance and hypertension, which are three crucial components of metabolic syndrome.

Excess Weight

Those who are overweight, especially those who are obese, are more prone to developing metabolic syndrome. The farther the person goes above the acceptable weight line, the more prone he or she becomes to developing this syndrome and the effects associated with it. Basic logic will dictate that the more excess weight a person has, the more fat will deposit at any single point of the body. Chances are, some of this fat will be deposited at the peritoneum. This being said, individual genetics play a large role in where a person's body fat will be stored on their body. Nonetheless, the higher your visceral fat, the more prone you are to developing this syndrome.

Physical Inactivity

Physical inactivity brought about by a sedentary lifestyle is directly linked to increased incidences of metabolic syndrome. Those who don't get much physical activity are more predisposed to accumulating visceral fat, lowered HDL cholesterol, and an increase in blood triglyceride and glucose levels. While increased awareness of the negative effects of sedentary living has been hammered on through various mediums, getting into an active lifestyle is simply not easy. Technological developments (ex. computers, elevators) have made it easier for people to live a "fulfilling" life while not having to be physically active.

Genetics

Metabolic syndrome and most of its associated conditions are mainly acquired through lifestyle choices. However, it cannot be discounted that genes do play a role in increasing one's chance of developing the syndrome. For example, some people are just more prone to developing diabetes and cardiovascular disease than others. Also, some ethnic groups are found to be at a higher risk of developing metabolic syndrome than others. For example, Hispanics and Asians are specifically singled out as at-risk races for developing this condition.

As a multifaceted health problem, a detailed multi-step approach is necessary to prevent the development of this all-too-common syndrome (for those who don't have it) and to reverse its effects (for those who have it). While the genetic factor may be discouraging to some, it is important to remember that we must focus on the factors that we can control, rather than sulking in the idea that we were dealt a poor hand.

Chapter 4:

The Complications of Metabolic Syndrome

For those who are not in the academe or the medical field, metabolic syndrome is one of the least-understood medical conditions in the world. However, it is a fast-rising disease that is starting to spread in pandemic proportions. As mentioned earlier, in the United States alone, roughly a third of the population has this syndrome, thus them prone to all kinds of potential health problems.

When not reversed, it can be said that such people are essentially ticking time bombs. Just to give you an idea of what a person is going up against, this chapter will take a closer look to the litany of health complications associated with metabolic syndrome.

Type 2 Diabetes

Diabetes mellitus is one of the most dangerous diseases in the modern world. Related to this, type 2 diabetes is considered a hallmark symptom associated with metabolic syndrome. For those who don't know, type 2 diabetes is actually caused by insulin resistance, in comparison to type 1 diabetes, which is mainly caused by insulin insufficiency.

Insulin resistance is triggered by the development of visceral fat, leading to all kinds of health issues. Peripheral nerve damage, retinopathy, kidney issues, and poor wound healing potentially leading to gangrene are just some of the complications associated with diabetes.

Atherosclerosis

This is one of the more common complications associated with metabolic syndrome. Basically, this is triggered by increased levels of triglycerides and cholesterol in the bloodstream, a common issue associated with obesity and chronic hyperglycemia. This is also brought about by a reduced level of HDL in the bloodstream, which causes the buildup of fat (plaque) on the arterial walls.

The problems caused by such accumulation are twofold: it reduces blood flow and it hardens the arterial walls. A myocardial infarction (heart attack) becomes the end result either because of cardiac ischemia (lack of blood flow to cardiac tissues) or a ruptured blood vessel (usually the coronaries).

Heart Disease

Heart disease often goes hand in hand with metabolic syndrome because of the many factors that makes someone with the syndrome an easy target for future heart failure. It has already been mentioned that atherosclerosis alone can cause a heart attack. Hypertension also plays a major role in the development of heart disease. Increased blood pressure can potentially cause the rupture of small and/or weakened blood vessels.

Furthermore, high blood pressure is also a sign that the heart is getting overworked. Chronic hypertension is linked to the development of just about every kind of cardiovascular disease, so the fact that metabolic syndrome is a risk factor for heart disease is fundamentally academic in nature.

Kidney Disease

A close association between metabolic syndrome and renal dysfunction has been uncovered. However, due to the complex relationships between these two conditions, it is not exactly clear what their true cause-and-effect relationship is. Still, it is easy to see why those with metabolic syndrome are expected to have kidney problems sooner or later.

Hypertension is known to cause damage to the kidneys, specifically the glomeruli. Additionally, diabetes can cause kidney damage due to chronic excess glucose filtration. Albuminuria (protein found in urine) and a lower glomerular filtration rate (GFR), primary indicators of compromised kidney function, are usually observed in patients with metabolic syndrome.

Nonalcoholic Fatty Liver Disease

The association between metabolic syndrome and the development of Nonalcoholic Fatty Liver Disease (NAFLD) is strong. Even though the cause-and-effect relationship between the two diseases is not yet fully identified, both health conditions have causative agents and predispositions connected to each other. Obesity, increased blood glucose and triglyceride levels, and physical inactivity are all linked to development of NAFLD.

At the same time, NAFLD contributes to the further development of metabolic syndrome because a fatty liver produces excess amounts of glucose and triglycerides. Liver failure may ensue due to cirrhosis, hepatitis and hepatic carcinoma caused by excess fat deposits.

Strokes

Also termed as a "brain attack," is one of the leading causes of death and disability in the modern age. Strokes, brain damage caused by circulatory impairments, are caused by a number of factors. A number of these factors, including impeded blood flow and aneurysms, are directly linked to the effects associated with metabolic syndrome.

Obesity, hypertension, and abnormal serum fat levels are all risk factors for developing a stroke. As such, it is easy to conclude that those with metabolic syndrome are at a higher risk of experiencing a stroke later in life.

Neurologic Disorders

It has been observed that people with metabolic syndrome are at a higher risk of developing neurologic disorders, such as depression and Alzheimer's disease. While the exact molecular mechanism for such an effect is not yet fully understood, there is evidence that proves that multiple cellular alterations caused by metabolic syndrome are linked to the development of neurologic disorders.

It has been hypothesized that the alterations to the levels of compounds, such as adipokines, cytokines, and hormones, are linked to the deterioration of nervous system function. Studies are still ongoing to uncover the full relationship between metabolic syndrome and neurologic disorders.

Needless to say, there are plenty of health implications connected to the emergence of metabolic syndrome. If left unchecked, this disorder can potentially harm or kill a person through various means. The good news is that the outlook for patients is still very good, as long as the symptoms associated with the disorder are properly handled. It is because of these reasons why a strong emphasis in preventing the rise of this disease has been made.

Chapter 5:

Ways to Diagnose Metabolic Syndrome

Treatment begins with diagnosis, as this helps in determining the issues that the patient must address as well as the potential means for management applicable for a given case. One interesting thing about diagnosing this condition is that not all medical authorities and organizations agree to the parameters used as basis for determining if a patient is positive for metabolic syndrome. However, for reference, we will try to discuss some of the methods and standards used for diagnosis.

Just for a review, here are the five fundamental criteria used in diagnosing metabolic syndrome. Being positive in at least three of these criteria means that you already have the condition. The more criteria that are applicable to you, the more severe your condition is and the more prone you become to developing health problems in the future. Some organizations include other standards for diagnosis, but these five are still considered as the "golden standard" for diagnosing metabolic syndrome.

Waist Circumference

Waist circumference, together with weight, is used to determine if a person is obese. Also, waist circumference serves as a basis for determining the amount of visceral fat present on the patient. While standards may vary according to race, the following values are generally accepted for diagnosing a patient with metabolic syndrome: above 40 inches for men and above 35 inches for women.

Blood Pressure

Chronic hypertension is one of the fundamental signs of metabolic syndrome. A person is determined to be hypertensive if his/her blood pressure readings are constantly at or above 140/90. Also, a patient is hypertensive if he/she is already receiving medications for controlling blood pressure.

Fasting Blood Sugar

This is the golden standard for diagnosing both metabolic syndrome and diabetes mellitus. If you have FBS levels above 100 mg/dl, then you are considered to be hyperglycemic. If the value is above 125 mg/dl, then you are at a higher risk as it means that you are diabetic and severely hyperglycemic.

Blood Triglyceride

Aside from being a risk factor for cardiovascular disease, the presence of excess triglycerides in your blood is an indicator of metabolic syndrome. If you have triglyceride levels above 200 mg/dl or you are taking medications for managing such levels, then you are considered to have abnormally high triglyceride levels.

HDL Levels

High-density lipoprotein levels have been recently used as a determinant of cardiovascular health. Known as "good cholesterol," having low levels of HDL is directly linked to the development of atherosclerosis. Men with lower than 40 mg/dl and women with lower than 50 mg/dl of HDL have low HDL, and they are at a higher risk of developing cardiovascular   problems.

If at least three of these criteria are applicable to you, then you most likely have metabolic syndrome. Aside from this, other health authorities make use of other standards for diagnosing patients. Here are just some of the world's biggest health organizations and their conditions on how to define and diagnose metabolic syndrome.

World Health Organization

The WHO mainly determines metabolic syndrome cases using two groups of evaluating data. You are positive for metabolic syndrome if:

You have any one of the following: diabetes mellitus, insulin resistance, and/or impaired glucose tolerance

You have any two of the following: hypertension, low HDL, high triglycerides, central obesity, and/or microalbuminuria.

American Heart Association

The AHA uses the five fundamental signs of metabolic syndrome as their sole basis for diagnosis. If you have at least three of them, then you are already positive of the syndrome, and it is advisable to seek for immediate treatment and management.

International Diabetes Foundation

The IDF defines metabolic syndrome as having central obesity and any two of the following: high triglycerides, low HDL, hypertension, and increased fasting plasma glucose. Body mass index can also be used for determining central obesity. The increased emphasis on central obesity is asserting the point that it is the most important criterion for defining metabolic syndrome.

There are a few other diagnostic techniques used in diagnosing metabolic syndrome. An example is the use of serum markers, such as high-sensitivity C-reactive protein. Used as a means for predicting coronary vascular diseases and nonalcoholic fatty liver disease, these markers can determine those prone to the common manifestations of metabolic syndrome. The presence of other health conditions (ex. polycystic ovary syndrome and lowered testosterone) is also useful for diagnostic evaluation. Other diagnostic effects are still under development as of this moment.

Chapter 6:

Prevention and Treatment Options

Because of the sheer prevalence of metabolic syndrome, it may give an impression that this epidemic is an unsolvable problem that will kill you softly until your body just gives out. However, this is certainly not the case. In fact, the outlook for people with metabolic syndrome is great, as long as proper care and treatment is administered as soon as possible.

At the same time, prevention is relatively simple for those who don't have it. As long as one takes care of his/her body well, the prospects are good for keeping metabolic syndrome at bay. Here is a list of some of the best prevention and treatment options out there.

Exercise

Physical activity is an effective antidote for a lot of the conditions involved in metabolic syndrome. First of all, it helps in burning off excess calories and fat stores, helping you lose excess weight and maintain an ideal physical composition. Also, it helps in improving cardiovascular health, strengthening the heart, and reducing blood pressure.

Regular physical activity also helps in building muscle, which can improve your physical fitness and metabolic rate. At least 30 minutes of moderate-intensity exercise decreases the risk of developing metabolic syndrome and dozens of other ailments.

Healthy Eating

Eating habits play an important role in our health. Practicing the right eating habits has a positive compound effect that will become self-sustainable. Likewise, poor eating habits dig us deeper into a position where we are forced to climb out of. For the sake of your health, you must follow healthy eating habits. Making sure you get the proper amount of micronutrients and macronutrients to support your daily endeavors is essential. To discover your basic micronutrient and macronutrient needs, see a nutritionist who will walk you through the process.

Weight Loss

Losing excess weight has a lot of positive effects on the human body. Reduction of excess weight helps in lowering blood pressure, regulating serum fat levels, improving the body's response to insulin, and reducing blood glucose levels.

Most importantly, weight loss helps in reducing visceral fat and all the pathological effects it causes. Losing weight is central to any plan of preventing metabolic syndrome and its associated diseases from taking a hold on one's body.

Quit Smoking

There is a wide range of scientific evidence supporting the stance that cigarette smoking is directly associated with the emergence of metabolic syndrome, such as causing hypertension.

While some people still consider this link as inconsistent or controversial, a positive correlation in a significantly high number of studies shows that an association between smoking and metabolic syndrome may not be all that farfetched. Even if it can be argued that such claims are inconclusive, when you consider its numerous health benefits, quitting smoking is a classic low-risk, high-reward step.

Medications

Your doctor may prescribe medication if some of the components of metabolic syndrome are deemed to be on the high-risk part of the spectrum. When prescribed, some of these drugs can help with managing these risk factors. When combined with other health habits, the use of medication can greatly help while the patient tries to manage his condition.

However, there is always the potential for side effects and interactions that can make prescription risky or impossible. Regardless of the case, for safety reasons, it is important for the patient to undergo screening before taking any specific medications.

By living a healthy lifestyle and keeping its components in check, you can fight metabolic syndrome. Most importantly, the implementation of the aforementioned techniques can prevent it from hitting you in the first place. While these tips may *seem* easy to do, they may not actually *be* easy not to do. Focus on creating habits rather than isolated occurrences.

Chapter 7:

The Future of Metabolic Syndrome

Metabolic syndrome is one of the most pressing health issues in most countries today, especially in the Western World. With so many people affected by it, the race is on to find a possible way to reduce its incidences. Considering that this condition is linked to all kinds of health problems, resolving it has a huge potential for reducing the incidences of diseases, such as coronary heart disease and type 2 diabetes, both locally and globally.

Reducing disease cases also reduces the strain on the medical workforce and reduces expenses spent on health care. Because of this fact, and the fact that it is a risk factor for a lot of illnesses, it is no surprise why policy makers are prioritizing efforts to prevent and reduce cases of metabolic syndrome.

As metabolic syndrome is largely considered to be a lifestyle-induced health problem, policy makers mainly target lifestyle changes as the way to reduce metabolic syndrome cases within families and communities. This is mainly done through health education, such as this through book. By increasing awareness of the pathologic effects of metabolic syndrome, the general public can perform preventive measures in their own homes. At the same time, promotion of healthy living practices and access to medical assistance help reduce cases of metabolic syndrome around the world.

Aside from shifting health care priorities, another thing that can affect the future of metabolic syndrome is the development of future treatment methods. One example of this is the creation of a prototypical drug called the Polypill. A theoretical combination of six different pharmacological compounds (aspirin, folic acid, three antihypertensives, and a statin), the aim of such a medication is to reduce the effects of both cardiovascular disease and metabolic syndrome.

However, the effects of the Polypill are still unproven, and the drug is still very much in its experimental stages. An alternative approach, the Polymeal, utilizes different foods to reduce the risk of cardiovascular disease.

The race for finding a feasible long-term solution for the metabolic syndrome problem is still very much on. With many people already dealing with its effects and more still prone to developing it, the medical community, scientists, researchers, entrepreneurs, and policy makers are in a race to find a lasting solution to this condition that leaves people from all walks of life prone to a "constellation of diseases."

Conclusion

Thank you for reading this! We hope this short, concise book was able to teach you a thing or two about metabolic syndrome.

While this book serves as a short overview to inform you on the essential issues and solutions regarding metabolic syndrome, you should seek a medical professional if you are looking for one-on-one advice tailored to your specific needs.

If you've learned anything from this book, please take the time to share your thoughts by sending me a personal message, or even posting a review on Amazon. It would be greatly appreciated and I try my best to get back to every message!

Thank you, and good luck in your journey to optimal health!

www.ingramcontent.com/pod-product-compliance
Lightning Source LLC
Chambersburg PA
CBHW072309200526
45168CB00014B/1182